KETOGENIC DIET

OVER 50+ QUICK AND EASY RECIPES TO LOSE WEIGHT, BURN YOUR BELLY FAT AND LIVE HEALTHY ON A LOW CARB DIET

INTRODUCTION

Everyone wants to live a healthy and fulfilled life through maintaining physical fitness, healthy eating, and mostly little or no visit to a hospital unless on checkup reasons. Did you know that Ketogenic diets (KD) were initially remedy and treatment for epilepsy? Come to think of it; if such food is so powerful to be used as a healing remedy, how much more if you consider it your daily diet? A Ketogenic diet has origin from the word ketosis which refers to a body state where the body utilizes body fat for energy due to reduced carbs levels which affects the amount of glucose in the body

The main reason for observing a KD is usually to lower the proportion intake of carbohydrates and increase fats intake in a meal. Dietary results related to fasting are directly the same as those that come with observing a Keto diet only that in fasting the body is deprived some very essential. People have used starvation as a weight-loss method without the knowledge of possible harms that it can cause the body. Not every nutrient is responsible for weight loss or an increase in body fat, so starvation is a quick fix that can lead to a health issue. The human body has fat and fat-free mass made of lean muscle, water, minerals and other nutrients. Now your goal here is to reduce what you have in excess instead of changing your body composition by starving yourself of all nutrients.

How does Ketogenic diets work

I.   Carbohydrates breakdown

A Carbohydrate molecule is composed of three elements carbon, hydrogen and oxygen. Different combinations of atoms from this elements form different types of carbohydrates and that is why when carbohydrates are mentioned you will hear other terminologies such as monosaccharides, glucose, polysaccharides, starch, cellulose, glycogen, disaccharides, fructose, Ribose and deoxyribose, galactose and polysaccharides. The name carbohydrate comes from its chemical composition 'carbo' and hydrate denoting carbon dioxide and water respectively

This carbohydrates have different functions depending on the organism and the conditions. When broken down in the presence of oxygen, carbohydrates release water, carbon dioxide and energy as a byproduct. The essential carb is glucose when it comes to the human body and the ketogenic diet specifically. The formula for glucose is quite simple $C_6H_{12}O_6$, during the breakdown of glucose, glucose will combine with oxygen ($C_6H_{12}O_6 + 6O_2 \rightarrow 6CO_2 + 6H_2O$) in the form of respiration known as glucose oxidation or reduction.

II.   Human Body energy requirements

The human body energy requirements are determined by a number of factors. Energy requirement can be determined by the energy expenditure through physical activities, energy need for growth, energy need for psychological functions. The brain is known to be the most energy-consuming organ in the body at around 20%. Other organs include the heart, kidneys, liver, lungs, and skeletal muscles, among others. Perhaps you might be getting the perception that conclusion to this material will be to use your brain more to lose more weight. Research has alternative facts concerning this matter and scientific research indicating that the brain is still active even when resting or sleeping. Regardless of the amount of energy one uses for brain functions, the main aim of this material is to ensure that there is no excessive glucose converted into fats. Excessive consumption of carbohydrates is the main focus of this material. A study carried out for six individuals over 10 days is a proof that when the bodies energy requirements are met by having the diet meet energy requirements only, there is no recorded significant weight gain. This has given birth to the Ketogenic diet whose primary function is to ensure that energy requirements are met without an unnecessary increase in body fat and consequently weight gain. In coming up with the recipes, the main goal is to ensure that energy requirements are met by utilizing stored fats and other nutrients balanced. Determining energy requirement is not a walk in the park for anyone from their houses; a combination of scientific calculations are used to determine energy requirements. However, research has various activities mapped out on the energy consumption of various body organs and the energy requirement for the whole body during some given activities.

First, to study various organs energy consumption, this is done when the subject is sleeping since when one awake various activities will change the energy consumption of various organs. The rate at which the body converts energy or rather consumes energy when one is sleeping is called the basal metabolic rate. This basal metabolic rate is not the same for everybody and therefore it is quite important for one to understand their body in order to understand how much energy one consumes at during sleep so as to establish the excess energy.

III.   Calculating basic metabolic Rate

Basal metabolic rate or rather as earlier stated the rate at which the body consumes energy during sleep. As body size increases, BMR also increases and the vice-versa is also true. Body size is measured in terms of weight, height and surface area. Therefore when trying to lose some weight calorie intake quite important since weight gain or weight loss also happens during sleep. There have been very many cases of people working out or engaged in very physical activity but still gaining weight, perhaps they should check their calorie intake, especially by establishing their BMR. Various methods of calculating BMR have been proposed with varying degrees of accuracy, the most accurate method is known as the **Mifflin-St Jeor Equation**

Mifflin-St Jeor Equation:
For men:

$$BMR = 10W + 6.25H - 5A + 5$$

For women:

$$BMR = 10W + 6.25H - 5A - 161$$

W is body weight in kg
H is body height in cm
A is age
F is body fat in percentage

Weight, height and age are quite easy to know, but the problem comes in when trying to establish body fat percentage. It's good to state that weight scales will give different results and therefore it is recommended that one takes weight measure at the same time of the day for several consistent days then get an average. Now you don't have to worry about these formulas. There are very many apps and online calculators where you only need to feed the data and then you get your BMR.

IV.   Calculating Body fat percentage

Perhaps you must have noticed that in the formula for measuring BMR (F) was not used. F is the represents body fat. Body fat is different from weight since weight can be attributed to muscles and other body components. It is also good to note that weight gain associated with increasing in body fat is not healthy after certain limits. To calculate body fat percentage the first thing is to get your body mass index calculated as $W \div (H)^2 \times 703$

After getting this figure, the next step is to calculate body fat percentage. Again the formula is different between men and women.

Women   (1.20 x BMI) + (0.23 x Age) - 5.4= Body Fat Percentage
Men (1.20 x BMI) + (0.23 x Age) - 16.2 = Body Fat Percentage

Now the first formula for calculating **BMR** does not consider body fat percentage and there are modified formula exists known as **Katch-McArdle Formula** calculated as follows

$$BMR = 370 + 21.6(1 - F) W$$

Apart from calculating **BMR** body fat percentage is important in determining if an individual has the recommended body fat. The chart below represents some recommended body percentages.

Body Fat Percentatge Calculation				
*Female : (1.20 x BMI) + (0.23 x Age) - 5.4 = Body Fat Percentage				
*Male : (1.20 x BMI) + (0.23 x Age) - 16.2 = Body Fat Percentage				
*BMI = W ÷ (H) 2 × 703				
Gender	Age	Under Fat	Healthy	Overweight	Obese
Female	20-40	<21%	21-33%	33-39%	>39%
Female	41-60	<23%	23-35%	35-40%	>40%
Female	61-79	<24%	24%-36%	36% to 42%	>42%
Male	20-40	<8%	8%-19%	19%-25%	>25%
Male	41-60	<11%	11-22%	22%-27%	>27%
Male	61-79	<13%	13-25%	25%-30%	>30%

V.   Ketosis

Ketosis is the process by which the liver produces chemicals called ketones that are required to burn fat for energy if the body does not have enough carbohydrates. We have gone through the process of determining if the carbs you are taking are enough, less than required or excess. We have also mentioned that excess carbohydrates will be converted into fats leading to fat accumulation and unhealthy weight gain. By using the formulas and available online calculators, you can know your energy requirements and the amount of fat you need to burn. Working out while still taking excess carbohydrates will lead to more weight and fat accumulation. Working out and exercising is not all about losing weight and burning fat but it goes beyond this to physical fitness, mental fitness, improving moods, better sleep, better sexual life, reducing doctor appointments, muscle and bones fitness and skin health among others. Now all this can be achieved, but you can still have extra weight and fat. To cure this, you need a ketogenic diet that will ensure that you are getting enough energy without storing unnecessary fats.

VI.   Low body fat percentage

In the chart above, we have given the recommended fat percentages for different ages and gender. There is a reason as to why there is a minimum recommended fat content. Since body fats make you gain weight or make you unhealthy, this does not call for total body fat elimination and that is why I strongly recommend that anyone who wants to go a ketogenic diet should first measure the fat percentage. Low body percentage can be equally harmful to your body. At this point is also important to note the difference between essential and stored fats. Essential fats are required for cellular processes as well as acting as reserve energy as well as keeping the body warm. Body fat also helps in cushioning internal organs from injury in case of an external impact as well as ensuring normal body process such as growth and immune building alongside women's reproductive health are going on as expected. Essential vitamins such as A, D, E and K can only be absorbed in the presence of fat. Vitamin A is responsible for good vision, a healthy immune system, reducing acne, strong bones growth and fertility. Vitamin D will maintain healthy bones, immunity, regulating insulin levels and cardiovascular health. Vitamin E has various benefits ranging from skin health, healing of wounds, skin itching, eczema, Psoriasis, fine lines wrinkles, as well as nail health. Finally, Vitamin K is responsible for bone health, cognitive health, heart health and helps in blood clotting. I think these are enough scares for anyone not to engage in the unplanned diet in the name of losing fat.

VII.   Calculating daily energy requirements

Now after having the energy requirements for the body at rest and also after calculating the percentage of body fat this is usually the first step towards setting your goals and determining on what to achieve. However, this has only factored in the energy requirements during sleep and body fat percentage. It's difficult or almost impossible to come up with a material or a formula that can universally calculate the energy requirements during the activity hours or rather when one is not sleeping. This is because every individual has different daily routine involving sitting, standing, walking, running, lifting, among other activities. When one engages in an activity that requires more energy than what he has consumed, the ketos concept kicks in where stored fat is utilized to give the body the required energy for the activity. So the answer as to why some people work out and will never lose weight is quite simple: they take more calories than they need for the particular activity and therefore the process of fat burning never starts and most cases more carbs will be converted into fats. To establish the amount of energy required during different activities there exist several tools available online that you need only to enter your weight and then you get the number of calories you can burn within a given duration to be able to plan your day. Therefore before engaging I any diet it advisable to know your body to be able to set targets.

VIII.   Signs that a Ketogenic diet is finally working

Many people would want immediate results when on a new diet or when they start working out. Unfortunately, that never happens and if you were to lose a lot of weight within a week, it could be an indication of some health problem. The Ketogenic diet is no exception, but what you don't know is that when you start a new workout routine or diet, the body adjusts and makes necessary metabolic changes to accommodate the new routine. Sometimes this process is not smooth and it could cause some pain. If you have ever been to a yoga or gym class, you will attest that the first few days are usually rough, especially when the instructor pushes you to go harder on the first few days. Here are some common signs that the Ketogenic diet is finally working.

a. Thirst and dry mouth

As earlier mentioned, glucose breakdown gives out energy carbon dioxide and some water molecules. When not taking your previous carbohydrates quantity, the water from glucose breakdown also reduces. Release of the ketones into the blood to burn fat for energy causes fluid and electrolyte imbalance in the cells. The only known danger of drinking too much water is sodium dilution. Many people don't take the recommended 2litres per day and perhaps this is the time you need to go back to that amount. Drinks low in carbs are also recommended at this point. Organic coconut water and a little more salt in your food can assist in this but all in all this is a good sign that the process has begun.

b. Muscle cramps and spasms

Fluid and electrolyte imbalance are the primary cause of muscle cramps and spasms. Electrolytes are responsible for carrying electrical signals in the body and imbalance will lead to conflicting messages to the muscles and other body organs. To remedy this, foods rich in calcium, magnesium and potassium are recommended.

c. Headaches

This also goes back to dehydration and electrons imbalance. This will usually last from a few days to a week. More water and <u>foods</u> that increase electrons is recommended but make sure they are within the keto diet.

d. Stomach upsets

Whenever there is a dietary change, the gastrointestinal system will be disrupted. It takes some time for the stomach to adjust to the higher fat content digestion and if left undigested more water will be required to expel the fat sometimes causing diarrhea. Cramping, bloating and constipation is other common symptoms experienced due to reduced fiber intake, which is essential for the movement of food in the stomach. When this kicks in, there is always the temptation to go for fiber supplements, laxatives and anti-diarrhea tablets. This might cause more problems like dependency, microbiome disruption and inflammation. Fiber supplements are known to be high in carbohydrates and therefore, the benefits of a Ketogenic diet may be delayed. These problems will last for a few days to a week, and it's a sign that the diet is finally working. Some dietary remedies exist such as nuts, seeds, cruciferous vegetables and greens. Staying hydrated is also an excellent remedy.

e. fatigue and general body weakness

Carbohydrates give a quick source of energy and are less complicated to breakdown as compared to fats. When one switches to a Ketogenic diet, the first few days will be characterized by a mismatch between energy expenditure and energy intake. However, this will last for only a few days for most people. It's good to know that fatigue is also a symptom of dehydration and insufficiency in some nutrients. After few days these symptoms will slowly disappear and you will experience more energy levels

f. Bad breath

Ketones leave the body through breathing and urine. A specific ketone called acetone is associated with this bad breath. A fruity smell is also experienced. The remedy to this is only increasing the number of times you brush your teeth and sometimes chewing sugarless gum.

g. Weight loss and increased energy

Perhaps you might have to wait for a little bit longer for this to happen but when this kicks in you have already started burning the extra fat. The first few days, some weight loss might be experienced, but this is only associated with water content decrease. The real weight loss occurs after several weeks, depending on the individual.

h. Sleep disruption

In the first few days, insomnia might kick in and or waking up in the night. This is associated with low levels of serotonin and melatonin in the keto diet. There is no need to remedy this since it will go away after a few days and deeper quality sleep will be experienced thereafter.

IX. Diseases whose symptoms can be treated by Ketogenic diet

It is worth noting that some of these conditions have overlapping symptoms and also some of these symptoms could indicate some other issues. The table below is not a guide to self-diagnosis but the emphasis should be on the reasoning behind the Ketogenic diet and how the diet will help in mitigating some of the symptoms. If you have any of these symptoms, it is advisable to see a doctor. The reasoning behind the dietary cure is the same used when making dietary supplements and medicines for various dietary-related ailments. Your body might not be able to absorb the required nutrients from the diet at first, so this diet does not call for abandoning your medications altogether. Medicines are quite expensive and the dependency on drugs has various side effects on the body. The main aim of this material is weight and fat percentage reductions and by regulating your weight, you also get to keep some of the lifestyle diseases away.

Disease	Symptoms		Why Ketogenic diet	
Epilepsy	I.	Temporary confusion	I.	Alternative to starvation
	II.	losing conscious and seizures	II.	Reduction of glutamate
	III.	Psychic signs	III.	Synthesis of GABA
	IV.	uncoordinated jerking movements	IV.	Brain inflammation reduction
Metabolic syndrome	I.	Large waist	I.	Glucose control
	II.	high levels of triglyceride,	II.	fat percentage reduction
	III.	high blood sugar,		
	IV.	high blood pressure		
Glycogen storage diseases	I.	Fatigue , Stunted growth and Gout	I.	Release of Ketones to burn fat as an alternative source of energy
	II.	Poor immunity		
	III.	Kidney and heart problems		
	IV.	Obesity and breathing problems		
	V.	Mouth sores and blood clotting problems		
Polycystic Ovary Syndrome (PCOS)	I.	Irregular periods and Heavy bleeding	I.	Reduction in insulin resistance
	II.	Hair growth, Acne and skin darkening	II.	Reduction in testosterone levels
	III.	Headaches		
	IV.	Infertility		
Diabetes	I.	Thirst, hunger and excessive urination	I.	Utilizing fats as an alternative source of energy
	II.	Fatigue, irritability and blurred vision		
	III.	Fruity and bad breath	II.	Controlling glucose carbohydrates levels
	IV.	Wounds		
	V.	Skin infections	III.	Reducing insulin requirements
Parkinson disease	I.	Stooped posture	I.	Helps in diminished mitochondrial energy metabolism
	II.	Cramped writing		
	III.	Slow movements as well as stiff limbs	II.	Reduction in alpha-synuclein
	IV.	Sleep disorder		
	V.	Voice changing		
GLUT1 Deficiency Syndrome	I.	Cognitive impairment	I.	Glucose energy alternative sources
	II.	Unclassified seizures		

	III. Myoclonic seizures	
	IV. Atonic seizures	
	V. Atypical seizures	
Multiple Sclerosis	I. Vision and cognitive problems	I. Reducing neurodegenerative component
	II. Fatigue	
	III. Balance and numbness issues	II. Oxidation stress reduction
	IV. Sexual dysfunction	
	V. Bladder problems	
Nonalcoholic Fatty Liver Disease	I. Fatigue	I. Fat reduction
	II. Jaundice	II. Insulin requirements and resistant reduction
	III. Red palms	
	IV. Enlarging blood vessels	III. Blood sugar control
	V. Abdominal and spleen swelling	
Alzheimer's Disease	I. Memory loss	I. An alternative for impaired glucose utilization
	II. Cognitive problems	
	III. Vision problems	II. Reducing insulin dependency
Migraine Headaches	I. Fatigue and dizziness	I. Anti-inflammation effect
	II. Nausea and vomiting	II. Reduced oxidation stress
	III. Dull headache developing into throbbing pain	III. Covering energy deficit in the brain
	IV. Loss of appetite and stomach upsets	IV. modulating cortical excitability

X.   Meal plan

Being on a restrictive diet can be hectic, boring, monotonous and hard to plan. Going back to the old diet is quite common which I can call some form of relapse. Diets sometimes will sometimes strain your budget. Whatever ingredients you have the main focus is to get enough energy and nutrients while at the same time minimizing carbs. Here is a sample meal plan that will ensure that belly fat will go.

Week 1			
	Breakfast	Lunch	Dinner
Monday	Easy Blender Pancakes	Cream Cheese Zucchini Spaghetti	Mustard Lemon Pork, Polenta & Green Beans
Tuesday	Wagon Wheel Sausage Pie	Bunless Burger	Zucchini Hash Browns
Wednesday	Sausage, Egg & Cheese	Asian Crack Slaw	Ham & Cheddar Wraps
Thursday	Green Breakfast Smoothie	Easy Cobb Salad	Buckeye Fat Bombs
Friday	Chocolate Peanut Butter Muffins	Chicken Zoodle Soup	Avocado Lime Salmon & Cauli-Rice
Saturday	Creamy Coffee Shake	Beef & Pumpkin Hash	Shrimp & Mushroom Zoodles
Sunday	Sausage Frittata	Chinese Beef Stir-Fry With Orange	Low Carb Chicken Quesadilla

Week 2			
	Breakfast	Lunch	Dinner
Monday	Creamy Scrambled Eggs	Avocado Lime Salmon & Cauli-Rice	Sriracha Lime Flank Steak
Tuesday	Corndog Muffins	Chicken & Mushrooms	Bunless Burger
Wednesday	Mini Crustless Quiches	BLT Avocado Wraps	Low Carb Chicken Quesadilla
Thursday	Easy Blender Pancakes	Shrimp & Mushroom Zoodles	Beef & Pumpkin Hash
Friday	Omelet With Pesto & Feta Cheese	Buckeye Fat Bombs	Cream Cheese Zucchini Spaghetti
Saturday	Green Breakfast Smoothie	Ham & Cheddar Wraps	Cheddar Chicken & Broccoli Casserole
Sunday	Wagon Wheel Sausage Pie	Zucchini Hash Browns	Beef Patties With Creamy Mustard

REFERENCES

- https://onlinelibrary.wiley.com/doi/full/10.1111/j.1528-1167.2008.01821.x

- https://news.harvard.edu/gazette/story/2012/05/unraveling-the-secrets-of-the-epilepsy-diet/

- https://www.webmd.com/drugs/2/drug-6000-8019/divalproex-oral/divalproex-sodium-enteric-coated-tablet-oral/details

- https://www.webmd.com/drugs/2/drug-1493-5/carbamazepine-oral/carbamazepine-oral/details

- https://pediatrics.aappublications.org/content/119/3/535

- https://www.healthline.com/nutrition/keto-diet-meal-plan-and-menu#shopping-list

- https://www.healthline.com/nutrition/15-conditions-benefit-ketogenic-diet#section8

- https://www.healthline.com/nutrition/ketogenic-diet-101#sample-meal-plan

- https://www.calculator.net/bmr-calculator.html
- https://www.gaiam.com/blogs/discover/how-to-calculate-your-ideal-body-fat-percentage
- https://www.nrv.gov.au/dietary-energy
- https://www.nrv.gov.au/dietary-energy
- https://basix.basixwellness.com/Tools_Energy_Activities
- https://opentextbc.ca/physicstestbook2/chapter/work-energy-and-power-in-humans/
- http://www.fao.org/3/y5686e/y5686e04.htm
- https://www.ncbi.nlm.nih.gov/pmc/articles/PMC6087750/
- https://www.ncbi.nlm.nih.gov/pmc/articles/PMC5485536/#CR16
- https://www.ncbi.nlm.nih.gov/pmc/articles/PMC5485536/
- http://large.stanford.edu/courses/2012/ph240/khan1/
- https://www.ncbi.nlm.nih.gov/pmc/articles/PMC6361831/
- https://www.ncbi.nlm.nih.gov/pmc/articles/PMC5322833/
- https://www.ncbi.nlm.nih.gov/pmc/articles/PMC5485536/#CR16
- https://www.doctorsbeyondmedicine.com/listing/foods-containing-electrons

XI.   KITCHEN ATTENTION

Every recipe contains some applicable rules to make sure it serves its purpose. Ketogenic recipes are not an exception and here are some of the compiled regulations you need to be careful to observe

i.   For a recipe that demands that you use an egg, it is usually recommendable if you choose a larger one. It may pose a challenge when you go for a smaller option and end up with a slight nutritionally affected meal.

ii.   When choosing to use protein powders that are low in carbs, then it is prudent to have either Isopura chocolate or Isopure vanilla.

iii.   Make sure that when it requires the use of almond milk, then the unsweetened one is to be in the ingredients.

iv.   You will notice that peanut or almond butter that are naturally prepared offer excellent results. The best way to excel in this will be by confirming that the composition of the ingredients do not exceed two items.

v.   Mozzarella cheese is effective when they are shredded, with low moisture and part-skim. You will not be able to get the best from fresh mozzarella.

vi.   Unless when preparing special meals; which are usually identified, you will notice that most recipes will be ready to be served ones. When a recipe is to be served for some couple of days, the instructions will always be clear. However, even the selective ones are usually recommended to be prepared mild to be for just one serving.

vii.   Choosing to include or not include some spices is entirely on you and may not really affect the nutrition of the meal. Some spices such as hot sauce, flakes, jalapeno peppers, and red peppers among others may not entirely affect your meal if not used.

viii.   When greasing the pans or the baking dishes, then you can use coconut oil, olive oil or avocado oil interchangeably. Do not use all of them together.

ix.   Spiralizer have proven to be of great benefit in these related meals. Acquiring one for yourself will make all the difference since many of the recipes will be possible to perform.

x.   Whenever you are using grounded beef, it must be prepared as 80% lean. It therefore requires that you make the adjustment when the beef you use happen to have fat content that may not measure with the appropriated earlier.

xi.   Finally, some recipe may be identified directly as sugar free or just abbreviated "SF".

XII.   ESSENTIALS IN KITCHEN

To accomplish ones task and deliver accurate meals, you need to get in hands some essential tools in your kitchen. Time consumed when preparing meals can be eliminated by you taking a step to acquire some relevant tools. Not only will the meals be accurate but there will be an element of creativity with what you bring on the dining table. While some tools in your kitchen are relevant during preparation, you may want to make sure that you invest in some of the following tools.

Spiralizer

Like mentioned earlier, I cannot over emphasize that you need to equip your kitchen with this tool to get the best keto meals results. It works magic on vegetables by making them in to noodles in a snap. You will find it very resourceful especially when preparing soups, low cabs pasta and many other dishes. Whether you need a single or multipurpose tool, your choice of the spiralizer is entirely on you. They come in options either as a hand held single purpose or a full size one that can give choices such as ribbons, thin or thick noodles and more to explore.

The Processor

A food processor will be in most of our kitchens. Just as essential as it is in other meals, so will you find it so in the preparation of Ketogenic meals. NutriBullet lists at the top of the available processors in the market. This has been facilitated by the fact the blending containers are multipurpose in using them as lids and also to-go containers. Most of the people find it comfortable to use them from anywhere. Cleaning them also comes with very minimal efforts.

Hand Mixer

Using manual mixers to beat an egg white has been outdated. That is why it is recommendable if you go for an electric hand mixer. It saves on the energy and time consumed in preparing some ingredients. The tool is speedy making mixing and beating a breeze.

Food Scale

Remember that you will be find most of the food may need the counting of calories and macros. As a result, it requires that you measure the quantity and ingredients that you will be using. This is where a food scale becomes very relevant.

REFERENCES

- https://www.tasteaholics.com/pdf/14-day-meal-plan.pdf?utm_campaign=mass-email&utm_source=email&utm_medium=newsletter
- https://www.myketocal.com/blog/top-five-kitchen-essentials-for-the-ketogenic-diet-chef/
- https://www.lowcarbspark.com/keto-kitchen-tools/

XIII.   KETO RECIPES

LOW CARB OATMEAL

Servings 1

Calories 453

Fat 36g

Proteins 18g

Carbs 15g

Fiber 10g

Sugar 1g

Ingredients

- ½ cup of water
- 2 tablespoons hemp hearts
- 2 tablespoons almond flour
- 2 tablespoons unsweetened shredded coconut
- 1 tablespoon golden flaxseed meal
- 1 tablespoon chia seeds
- ¼ teaspoon sweetener
- 1 pinch salt
- ½ teaspoon pure vanilla extract

Direction

i. Take a pot and place on a stove and heating it over low heat. Add the ingredients to the saucepan but do not use the vanilla yet

ii. Constantly stir them while they cook for 3 to 5 minutes to that to achieve a thickened solution. Finally, add the vanilla and stir for a few minutes.

iii. Remove from the saucepan and serve while it is still warm.

CHOCOLATE PROTEIN SHAKE

Servings 1

Calories 440

Fat 31g

Proteins 15.6g

Carbs 8.2g

Ingredients

- ¾ cup almond milk
- ½ cup ice
- 2 tablespoon almond butter
- 2 tablespoon unsweetened cocoa powder
- 2 to 3 tablespoon Keto friendly sugar substitute
- 1 tablespoon chia seed
- 2 tablespoon hemp seeds
- 1 tablespoon pure vanilla extract
- Pinch kosher salt

Direction

i. Take the blender and add the ingredients in it except the chia and hemp.

ii. Blend them at a low speed increasing up to high speed for relatively 5 minutes or until you attain a smooth solution.

iii. Serve the smoothie into a glass and use the hemp and chia seed to garnish.

iv. Enjoy it with a straw!

SHRIMP & MUSHROOM ZOODLES

Servings 3

Calories: 500

Fats 32g

Proteins 44g

Carbs 7.5g

Ingredients

- 1 Tablespoon olive oil

- 8 Ounces white mushrooms, sliced

- 1 Tablespoon butter

- 6 Ounces jumbo shrimp, peeled

- 1 Large zucchini

- ¼ Cup marinara sauce

- Salt, pepper

- 2 Tablespoon parmesan cheese

Directions

i.   Firstly, take a large pan and pour olive oil in it. Allow it to heat over medium temperature.

ii.   Fry the mushrooms until they have soaked up most of the oil.

iii.   Add butter to the pan and allow the mushrooms to cook so that they turn golden.

iv.   Adding shrimp to the pan, cook each side for 4 minutes.

v.   Use the spiralizer to prepare zoodles separate as the shrimp continue to cook.

vi.   After the shrimp are cooked and turns pinkish, it is the time to add zoodles then cook for about 2 minutes.

vii.   The next thing will be to add marinara sauce then seasoning the meal with salt and pepper.

viii.   Enjoy with a sprinkle of parmesan cheese especially as a dinner meal.

https://www.tasteaholics.com/pdf/14-day-meal-plan.pdf?utm_campaign=mass-email&utm_source=email&utm_medium=newsletter

CHEDDAR CHICKEN & BROCCOLI CASSEROLE

Servings 4

Calories: 548

Fat 42g

Protein 44g

Carbs 4g

Ingredients

- 20 Ounces of chicken breast, shredded

- 2 Cups of broccoli florets, frozen is okay too

- 2 Tablespoon of olive oil

- ½ Cup sour cream

- ½ Cup heavy cream

- Salt, pepper

- 1 Teaspoon of oregano

- 1 Cup cheddar cheese, shredded

- 1 Ounce of pork rinds, crushed

Directions

i. Prepare the oven first by preheating it until it is 450 degrees Fahrenheit hot.

ii. Use a mixing bowl deep enough and put chicken, broccoli florets, sour cream and olive oil for mixing. Make sure it is done thoroughly.

iii. Grease an 8" by 11" baking dish then place your mixture then press it carefully to an even layer.

iv. Take the heavy cream and drizzle it on the layer uniformly. Add pepper, salt, and oregano for seasoning.

v.   Spread the cheddar cheese on top followed by pork rinds to form a crispy casserole topping.

vi.   Place the mix in the oven and bake it for not more than 25 minutes.

vii.   A ¼ of casserole is enough for a single meal and enough for nutritious lunch.

https://www.ketodietyum.com/keto-chicken-broccoli-casserole-with-cheddar-topping/

CREAMY SCRAMBLED EGGS

Servings 2

Calories: 710

Fats 57g

Proteins 37g

Carbs 2.5g

Ingredients

- 4 Large eggs

- 2 Tablespoons of butter

- 4 Strips bacon

- 2 Tablespoon of sour cream

- ½ Teaspoon of salt

- ¼ Teaspoon of black pepper

- 1 Stalk green onion

Directions

i.   Place a pan on a medium heated cooker, crack the eggs then add butter. Use a silicone spatula to stir continuously.

ii.   At the same time, be cooking some bacon strips in a different pan. Alternatively, you can bake them.

iii.   For best result stir the eggs while on the heat and off with intervals of 30 seconds. When almost done, turn off the heat then allow the eggs to cook with the residual heat in the pan.

iv.   Use the tablespoon of sour cream to top the egg and then use pepper and salt to season.

v.   Take the chopped green onions to garnish the meal.

vi.   It is best enjoyed when served as a breakfast meal.

https://www.tasteaholics.com/pdf/14-day-meal-plan.pdf?utm_campaign=mass-email&utm_source=email&utm_medium=newsletter

CHICKEN ZOODLE SOUP

Servings 3

Calories: 370

Fat 26g,

Proteins 23g

Carbs 8g

Ingredients

- 2 Tablespoons of olive oil

- ½ White onion, chopped

- 1 Medium carrot, chopped

- 1 Stalk celery, chopped

- 1 Tablespoon dried oregano

- 1 Quart chicken broth

- 8 Ounces of boneless, skinless chicken thighs

- 1 Large zucchini

- ¼ Cup of sour cream

Directions

i. Use a soup pot to heat the olive oil with medium heat then add onions. Cook them until they are translucent.

ii. Pour the chopped carrot and celery and use pepper, salt, and oregano to season. Continue cooking until they soften.

iii. Add chicken broth to the mixture and cook until they boil. Lower the heat to allow simmering and add the chicken then cook for 30 minutes.

iv. Use spiralizer to make the zucchini to thin noodles then add to the soup at the last few minutes, preferably 2 or 3 minutes.

v. Enjoy the soup combined with sour cream.

vi. The recipe can be served as three meals for nutrition purpose.

https://www.tasteaholics.com/pdf/14-day-meal-plan.pdf?utm_campaign=mass-email&utm_source=email&utm_medium=newsletter

CHOCOLATE PEANUT BUTTER MUFFINS

Servings 18

Calories 270

Fat 13g

Carbohydrates 37g

Protein 6g

Ingredients

- 1 Cup almond flour
- ½ Cup erythritol
- 1 Teaspoon baking powder
- 1 Pinch salt
- 1/3 Cup peanut butter
- 1/3 Cup almond milk
- 2 Large eggs
- ½ Cup SF chocolate chips

Directions

i. Excluding the chocolate, take all the dry ingredients and mix them in a mixing bowl then stir thoroughly.

ii. Take the almond milk and peanut butter, add to the mixture and stir to combine.

iii. As you mix, add one egg and stir it ultimately then add the other egg.

iv. Carefully fold the mix in the chocolate chips.

v. Use a muffin tin and add the mixture to the spaces. Bake for 15 minutes in an oven, making sure that it is at 350 degrees Fahrenheit.

vi. With these measures, you will get at least 6 muffins.

vii.   The nutrition value is in every 2 muffins served. It makes it a breakfast meal for three meals.

https://www.verybestbaking.com/recipes/143649/peanut-butter-chocolate-chip-muffins

CREAMY COFFEE SHAKE

Servings 1

Calories: 425

Fats 38g

Proteins 25g

Carbs 1g

Ingredients

- 1 Cup brewed coffee

- ¼ Cup heavy cream

- 1 Tablespoon coconut oil

- 1 Scoop vanilla protein powder approximately 30 grams

Directions

i.   Using a Nutribullet or a blender, add hot brewed coffee

ii.   Take the heavy cream, the coconut oil, and the protein powder and add to the blender.

iii.   Blend the mixture on high speed for 20 seconds.

iv.   Open the blender carefully to avoid burnings from steam created by the hot coffee.

v.   Enjoy it while still warm.

CLASSIC STEAK & EGGS

Servings 1

Calories: 687

Fats 52F,

Proteins 43P,

Carbs 5

Ingredients

- 1 Tablespoon olive oil

- 4 Ounces of sirloin

- 1 Tablespoon of butter

- 3 Large eggs

- Salt, pepper

- ½ Avocado

Directions

i. Using a pan, cook the sirloin until well done or desired doneness.

ii. On another pan, melt the butter then cook the two eggs while the yolk is still intact. Cook the yolk to the way you desire it done. Use salt and pepper to season.

iii. Take the sirloin and slice to preferred sizes then season with salt and pepper.

iv. Slice the avocado into small sizes and add some salt on the avocado.

v. Serve them together and enjoy a healthy breakfast.

https://www.tasteaholics.com/recipes/breakfast-recipes/steak-and-eggs/

PEPPERONI PIZZA OMELETTE

Servings 1-2

Calories: 600,

Fats 53

Proteins 32

Carbs 5

Ingredients

- 3 Large eggs
- 1 Tablespoon heavy cream
- ½ Ounces pepperoni slices
- ½ Cup shredded mozzarella
- Salt, pepper, basil.
- 2 Strips of bacon

Directions

i. Using the medium heated pan, add some oil moderately. On a side pan, have the bacon strips cooking.

ii. Crack the eggs in a bowl and bit them thoroughly mixing them with heavy cream. Pour them in the hot pan and allow them to cook to the point that they are almost done. You can add pepperoni slices on the sides.

iii. Take the mozzarella cheese then sprinkle it on the top of pepperoni then use salt, pepper, and basil to season and fold the omelette over.

iv. Continue cooking for about a minute then serve with bacon on the side.

https://www.tasteaholics.com/pdf/14-day-meal-plan.pdf?utm_campaign=mass-email&utm_source=email&utm_medium=newsletter

GREEN BREAKFAST SMOOTHIE

Servings 1
Calories 380
Fat 34g
Sodium 223mg
Potassium 753mg
Carbohydrates 12g
Fiber 8g

Sugar 3g
Protein 8g
Vitamin A 3085IU
Vitamin C 16.3mg
Calcium 314mg
Iron 3.1mg

Ingredients

1.5 Cup almond milk

1 Ounce spinach

50 Grams avocado

1 Tablespoon coconut oil

10 Drops liquid stevia

1 Scoop vanilla protein powder about 30 grams

Directions

Take all the ingredients listed and add them into the blender or use a Nutribullet.

Start blending slowly until you attain high-speed blending so that you acquire a

smooth and creamy solution.

Enjoy it as a morning smoothie breakfast.

https://www.tasteaholics.com/pdf/14-day-meal-plan.pdf?utm_campaign=mass-email&utm_source=email&utm_medium=newsletter

EASY BLENDER PANCAKES

Calories: 450,

Fats 29

Proteins 41

Carbs 4

Ingredients

- 2 Ounces cream cheese
- 2 Large eggs
- 1 Scoop vanilla protein powder about 30 grams
- 1 Dash cinnamon
- 10 Drops Liquid stevia optional
- 1 Pinch salt

Directions

i.   Put the ingredients to a blender then use high speed to attain a smooth and creamy solution.

ii. Place the griddle on a medium heat then spread the pancake batter in an even diameter.

iii. Cook each of the pancakes to a point where you see the bubbles forming, and the edges are a bit dry before flipping.

iv. Let the flipped pancake cook for few seconds and repeat the process until the mixture is ultimately used up.

v.   You may need some butter and drizzle sugar-free maple syrup to enjoy your pancakes fully.

https://www.tasteaholics.com/recipes/quick-bites/low-carb-pancakes/

SAUSAGE, EGG & CHEESE

Servings 1

Calories: 574,

Fats 49,

Protein 27

Carbs 1

Ingredients

- 3 Ounces breakfast sausage

- 1 Large egg

- 1 Tablespoon olive oil

- 1 Slice cheddar cheese

- Chives or green onion for garnish

Directions

i. Lightly oil the pan and place it on the heater then cook both the sausage and the egg. Make sure the sunny side is up or is over smooth.

ii. Take a slice of cheddar and arrange them with it then drizzle some hot sauce moderately if you want.

iii. Use the green onions and chives on top as garnish.

https://www.tasteaholics.com/pdf/14-day-meal-plan.pdf?utm_campaign=mass-email&utm_source=email&utm_medium=newsletter

HAM & CHEDDAR WRAPS

Servings 1

Calories: 600,

Fat 44g,

Protein 27g,

Carbs 8g

Ingredients

- 1 low carb wrap

- 2 tablespoon mayonnaise

- 2 ounces cheddar grated

- 2 ounces sliced ham

- Pickles or jalapenos to taste thinly sliced

- Salt and pepper

Directions

i. Take the skillet and heat it on a medium temperature then place the wrap on it so that it warms for about 30 seconds.

ii. Spread the mayonnaise on the wrap after it is warm as needed.

iii. Use the ham slices to place on top the take the grated cheese and sprinkle on top.

iv. Add the pickles and the jalapenos depending on your taste.

v. Season with pepper and salt then fold the ends to the inside and tightly make the role.

https://www.ketodietyum.com/keto-ham-cheddar-wraps/

BLT AVOCADO WRAPS

Servings 5

Calories: 640,

Fats 56

Proteins 18

Carbs 6

Ingredients

5 thick sliced turkey breast meat

Lettuce

Tomato slices

½ of an avocado

3 tablespoon fat-free mayonnaise

5 fully cooked bacon slices

Toothpicks

Directions

Place the avocado and mayonnaise in a mixing bowl and combine by mashing with a fork. You may blend them if you prefer smoother results.

Lay the turkey breast slice on a flat surface then spread a thin layer of the avocado mix at the centre, forming a circular spread.

Use one slice of the precooked bacon and place it at the centre of the slice.

Place the lettuce and the sliced tomatoes on top.

Take the turkey slice and gently roll it so that the fillings are inside the role then secure it at the centre with a toothpick.

Enjoy it as a nutritious lunch meal.

https://kimspireddiy.com/weight-watchers-lunches-best-ww-recipe-blt-avocado-turkey-wraps-with-smart-points/

EASY COBB SALAD

Serving Size: 2

Calories: 296

Fat: 11.2g

Carbohydrates: 10.6g

Protein: 38.5g

Ingredients

- 2 boneless, skinless chicken breasts

- 2½ cups spinach

- 2 hard-boiled eggs

- 4 pieces of cooked bacon

- 8 cherry tomatoes, sliced

- ¼ small chopped red onion

- ¼ cup bleu cheese

- Juice of 1 lime

- Sea salt and pepper to taste

Directions

i. Preheat the oven to 350 degrees in preparation for the cooking of the chicken.

ii. Line a parchment paper on a baking sheet then sprinkle salt and pepper as per your preference.

iii. Place the chicken in the oven to cook for 30 minutes. You can also use the temperature lowering to 165 degrees as a measure for the cooking.

iv. Prepare a bowl where you will put the mixture of salad one item at a time. Add to it spinach, sliced chicken, romaine, sliced tomatoes, bacon, chopped onions, eggs, and bleu cheese.

v. Drizzle lime juice to it and sprinkle the salt and pepper to season.

vi. You can choose to toss to combine or present it for service during lunch or dinner.

https://perfectketo.com/delicious-keto-cobb-salad/

ASIAN CRACK SLAW

Servings 6

Calories: 370

Fats 27

Proteins 24

Carbs 4

Ingredients

- 1 pound ground beef
- 1 garlic clove pressed
- 1 tablespoon sesame oil
- 9 ounces bag shredded cabbage
- 12 ounces bag broccoli slaw
- 2 teaspoon soy sauce
- 2 tablespoon BBQ sauce
- Salt and pepper to taste

Directions

i. Heat skillet in a medium-high heat then cook the beef until it attains the brown look. Use pepper and salt to season then transfer to a bowl or a plate as per your preference leaving the juice in the skillet.

ii. Use the juice left in the skillet to add garlic and cook for about approximately one minute.

iii. Add to it cabbage and the broccoli then cook to your desired tenderness.

iv. Add back the cooked beef to the mix.

v. Stir well while adding the soy sauce and BBQ sauce until the meal attains desirable heat all through.

vi. Mix with sesame oil.

vii. The Asian meal is ready for intake, especially for lunch hours.

https://www.lowcarbingasian.com/asian-crackslaw/

CHICKEN & MUSHROOMS

Servings 1

Calories 447

Fat 31g

Net carbs 1g

Protein 37g

Ingredients

- ¼ cup butter

- 2 cups sliced mushrooms

- Four chicken thighs

- ½ teaspoon onion powder

- ½ teaspoon garlic powder

- 1 teaspoon kosher salt

- ¼ teaspoon black pepper

- ½ cup of water

- 1 teaspoon alcohol-free mustard

- 1 tablespoon fresh tarragon

Directions

i. Use pepper, salt, garlic, and onion powder to season the chicken thighs.

ii. Use a heavy sauté pan to melt the one tablespoon of butter.

iii. Sear the thighs on the pan until they turn golden brown on each side for about four minutes each then removes them from the container.

iv. Melt the remaining butter on the pan. Cook the mushroom it for about four minutes until they attain golden brown appearance.

v. Deglaze the pan by adding water and the mustard.

vi. Place the chicken thighs back to the pan, making sure that the skin side is up.

vii. Use a cover and allow the chicken to simmer for relatively 15 minutes to ensure thorough cooking.

viii. Use the fresh tarragon to stir the meal and allow it to rest for about five minutes.

ix. Serve the meal while still hot for a lunch or dinner date.

https://www.ibreatheimhungry.com/skillet-chicken-mushrooms-low-carb-gluten-free-2/\

LOW CARB CHICKEN QUESADILLA

Servings 2
Calories 406
Fat 25.6g
Carbohydrates 5.2g
Fiber 2.6g
Protein 28.6g

Ingredients

- 2 tablespoons avocado oil

- 2 boneless skinless chicken thighs (Chop in ½inch pieces)

- 1 tablespoon taco seasoning

- ½ medium green chopped pepper

- 1 medium green onions sliced

- Salt and pepper

- 2 packs pizza crusts

- 1½ cups shredded cheese

Directions

i. Heat avocado oil in a medium heated skillet until shimmering and avoid smoking hot results. Cook the chicken and sauté for about five minutes then add the taco sparingly.

ii. To the mixture, add pepper and onions then cook to the point of attaining veggies tenderness. That should be relatively 3 to five minutes.

iii. Add one pack of the pizza crust then take the shredded cheese and sprinkle at least half cup of it.

iv. Spread half of the chicken fillings over the cheese then sprinkle about ¼ cup of the cheese again and lay the remaining pizza crust on top.

v. Cover the pan and allow the meal to cook for two to three minutes, maintaining the original heat. Repeat the process after flipping to the other side for two minutes only.

vi. Remove the skillet from the heat but allow the meal to continue cooking for a few minutes before slicing and serving.

vii. Repeat the process of cheese, crusts, and fillings with the remaining portions.

viii. The ingredients can prepare **Chicken Quesadilla** for four servings.

https://alldayidreamaboutfood.com/keto-chicken-quesadillas/

SRIRACHA LIME FLANK STEAK

Servings 6

Calories 398

Total Fat 27g

Saturated Fat 6g

Trans Fat 0g

Unsaturated Fat 19g

Cholesterol 90mg

Sodium 456mg

Carbohydrates 5g

Fiber 1g

Sugar 1g

Protein 32g

Ingredients

- 1½ pounds flank steak
- 1 teaspoon sea salt
- 1 teaspoon pepper, freshly cracked
- ½ cup olive oil
- 1 teaspoon Italian herb mix
- ¼ cup diced garlic
- 2 ounces lemon juice
- 1 tablespoon garlic powder
- Zest of 1 lemon

Directions

i. Place the steak on a flat surface in order to trim off any extra silver skin or fat on it.

ii. Use the pepper and salt to season it well and generously.

iii. Take a large bowl and put in olive oil, lemon zest plus juice, herbs, and the diced garlic then mix them thoroughly. Preferably you can also use a large plastic bag.

iv. Place the steak in the mixture and allow it to marinate for about 40 minutes and maximum for two hours.

v. Prepare your grill and allow it to heat to as high as 400 degrees Fahrenheit.

vi. Take the steak from the mixture and sprinkle the garlic powder on it.

vii. Transfer the steak on the hot grill making sure that you turn it every 4 to 5 minutes when cooking. Use some oil to wipe on the grill before placing the steak.

viii. Cook the steak to your preference where medium made is for about 10 minutes and well done for more minutes.

ix. Once it is done to your requirement, transfer the steak to a plate having folded it in a piece of foil and allow it carryover cooking for about ten minutes.

x. The steak should be ready to be sliced in to thin strips for service.

xi. Enjoy the meal while it is still hot with some veggies on the side.

https://sweetcsdesigns.com/the-best-garlic-grilled-flank-steak-recipe/

BUNLESS BURGER

Servings 2	Saturated Fat: 9g	Sugar: 1g
Calories: 318kcal	Cholesterol: 121mg	Vitamin A: 60IU
Carbohydrates: 3g	Sodium: 412mg	Vitamin C: 2.1mg
Protein: 21g	Potassium: 373mg	Calcium: 33mg
Fat: 23g	Fiber: 0g	Iron: 2.5mg

Ingredients

- 1 pound ground beef
- 1 egg
- 1 teaspoon mustard
- 1 teaspoon Worcestershire sauce
- 1 small onion grated
- ½ teaspoon garlic powder
- ½ teaspoon salt
- ½ teaspoon pepper
- ¼ teaspoon smoked paprika

Directions

i. Prepare the grill by lighting, cleaning, and oiling it.

ii. Use grated oil to extract its liquid using a dish towel so that it can be used as a marinade.

iii. Take the other ingredient and place them in a large bowl where you can use your hand to mix them thoroughly.

iv. Prepare some patties from the mixture and then use the thumb to form a shallow indent in each of them.

v. Use the grill to cool the burgers for 5 minutes or so that they are well done to your preference.

vi. Take a clean plate and place the burgers on them from the grill.

vii. Serve them together with some lettuce, tomatoes, red onions, and other preferable toppings.

https://www.thelittlepine.com/bunless-burger/

MUSTARD LEMON PORK, POLENTA & GREEN BEANS

Servings 4
Calories 729
Net carbs: (6 g)
Fiber: 3 g
Fat: (62 g)
Protein: 36 g

Ingredients

- 4 pork chops

- 2 tablespoon wholegrain mustard

- 1 tablespoon vegetable or olive oil

- 1 chicken bouillon cube

- ½ cup instant polenta

- ¼ cup cream

- ½ cup grated parmesan

- 3 tablespoon finely chopped flat-leaf parsley

- 10 ounces frozen green beans

- Lemon wedges

Directions

i. Use the mustard to rub the pork chops one side at a time and season. Prepare a frying pan and heat oil in it with a moderate temperature then cook the pork for 3 minutes or until it turns brown. Place it on a plate, cover with foil and rest it for five minutes.

ii. Take a saucepan and in moderate heat cook the crumbled bouillon cube using 1 cup of water.

iii. Place the polenta into the pan and cook it in moderate heat, whisking it to mix until it is well-cooked for about five minutes. You will tell it is cooked when it no longer sticks to the sides of the pan.

iv. Cook the beans in the microwave at a high temperature for three minutes or until you can tell they are well heated.

v. Add the beans, polenta, extra parsley and lemon wedges to the earlier served pork.

http://recipes-plus.com/recipe/mustard-pork-chops-polenta-green-beans-20888

AVOCADO LIME SALMON & CAULI-RICE

Servings 2

Calories per serving 420

Fat 127 g

Carbs 5g

Protein 37 g

Ingredients

- 50 grams cauliflower
- ½ avocado
- ½ lime
- 1 tablespoon red onion, diced
- 16 ounces salmon fillet
- Salt and pepper for tasting

Directions

i. Place the cauliflower into a processor and rice it then cooks it in a pan lightly heated and oiled for 8 minutes.

ii. Blend the lime juice, avocado and red onion when diced until it forms a smooth and creamy solution.

iii. Take the salmon and cook it in a skillet for 4 to 5 minutes each side starting with the skin side first (If you do not like salmon, substitute it with chicken thighs).

iv. Use a plate and lay a bed of cauliflower then serve the meal on it then generously pour the avocado solution prepared earlier.

https://www.tasteaholics.com/pdf/14-day-meal-plan.pdf?utm_campaign=mass-email&utm_source=email&utm_medium=newsletter

BUCKEYE FAT BOMBS

Calories: 301kcal

2g Net Carbs

3g Total Carbs

1g Fiber

9g Fat

1g Protein

1 Glycemic Load

Ingredients

- 8 ounces of cream cheese
- ½ cup peanut butter
- ¼ cup of coconut oil
- ¼ teaspoon kosher salt
- 2 teaspoons coconut oil
- 9 ounces of lily's chocolate chips

Directions

i. Take sheet pan and prepare by lining it with a silicon mat or an alternative of parchment paper then lay it aside.

ii. Take a bowl and put in it cheese, ½ cup of peanut butter, ¼ cup of coconut oil plus salt and mix thoroughly with a hand mixer or other kitchen aid you have. Ensure that you use medium speed when using a blender until you attain a fluffy and light solution.

iii. Put the bowl in a freezer for 10 to 15 minutes or in a fridge for one hour so that it can stiffen.

iv. Use a cookie scoop to make cookie balls on the sheet you prepared earlier. Make enough portions then place the sheet into the fridge for 5 minutes so that they can set up.

v. Melt the chocolate using the microwave, making sure you stir every 30 seconds while heating until it completely melts.

vi. Roll the peanut butter balls on your hands, make sure they are smoothly done.

vii. Take each at a time and deep them into the chocolate so that it covers ¾ of each.

viii. Use a parchment paper to line a clean sheet pan then place the balls on it. Use up all the mixture.

ix. Once done, place them in the fridge for about 10 minutes and they will be ready for eating.

https://www.midgetmomma.com/keto-buckeye-fat-bombs/

CREAM CHEESE ZUCCHINI SPAGHETTI

Servings
Calories 339
Fat 24g
Cholesterol 77mg
Carbohydrates 12g
Fiber 3g
Sugar 9g

Protein 21g

Ingredients

- 1 pound ground beef
- 15 ounces marinara sauce
- 4 ounces cream cheese
- 4 ounces sour cream
- 8 zucchini

Directions

i. Cook the beef on medium heat, making sure that you break it as it cooks to your preference then drain the fat.

ii. Use the marinara sauce and add it to the skillet together with the beef and heat it with medium temperature.

iii. Add the cheese and sour cream stir until they melt and are creamy then lower the heat. Cover the pan and allow the meal to simmer.

iv. Cut off the ends of the zucchinis and use the spiralizer to make noodles with them.

v. Using a different skillet, place it on the high heat and use a non-cooking spray on it.

vi. Cook the zoodles in it and tossing them over until they attain the texture that is preferable to you. Cook them in batches for about 3 minutes to ensure they do not release a lot of water.

vii. Serve the zoodles to a plate and top with the sauce and enjoy a delicious meal.

https://www.bunsinmyoven.com/low-carb-cream-cheese-zucchini-spaghetti/

OMELET WITH PESTO & FETA CHEESE

Servings 1

Calories 570

Fat 46g

Protein 30g

Carbs 2.5g

Ingredients

- 3 eggs
- 1 tablespoon butter
- 1 tablespoon heavy cream
- 1 ounce of feta cheese
- 1 tablespoon pesto
- Salt and pepper to taste

Directions

i. Put the eggs and heavy cream in a bowl and whisk them thoroughly.

ii. Melt the butter in a skillet placed on a medium heat then pour the mixture to cook until done.

iii. Use the cheese to crumble half of the omelette then spread the pesto over the cheese.

iv. Fold over the omelette and cook for 4 to five minutes so that the cheese melts well.

v. Use the remaining feta and some fresh herbs to serve.

https://www.ketodietyum.com/keto-omelet-with-pesto-feta-cheese/

SAUSAGE FRITTATA

Servings 4

Calories 655

Fat 42g

Proteins 33g

Carbs 32g

Fiber 6g

Sugar 8g

Ingredients

- 6 pork sausages
- 500g new potatoes
- 1 tablespoon olive oil
- 2 red onions, medium size, sliced
- 125 grams cheddar cheese, grated
- 6 large eggs
- 1-2 tablespoon wholegrain mustard

Directions

i. Heat the grill hot then cook the sausage while turning sides for about 8 minutes or until they attain golden color. Later slice so that each slice is thick enough.

ii. Chop the potatoes into chunks of roughly 1.5cm then boil them in water in a medium-size pan until they are tender.

iii. Heat the red onion in a heavy-based cooking pan for about 5 minutes until they soften. Take the potatoes, drain them and cook them in the pan for 2 to 3 minutes tossing them to mix with the onions. Use pepper to season then add the sausage slices and continue tossing them until they mix well.

iv. Tale the eggs and beat them then pour into the pan and use a wooden spoon to swirl the mixture so that to attain evenly covered filling for about 3 minutes.

v. Take the pan and place it on the grill then cook for another 3 minutes.

vi. Remove the pan and allow them to stand for a few minutes.

vii. Serve the meal with some mixed salad on the side.

https://www.sainsburysmagazine.co.uk/recipes/one-pot/sausage-frittata-with-mustard

BEEF PATTIES WITH CREAMY MUSTARD SAUCE

Servings 3

Calories 509

Fat 24g

Proteins 39g

Carbs 5g

Fiber 0g

Ingredients

- 500g ground beef
- ½ tablespoon butter
- 1 tablespoon olive oil
- 1 spring onion chopped
- 2 cloves garlic minced
- 100g mushrooms, thinly sliced
- Salt and pepper to taste
- Mustard cream sauce
- ½ cup heavy cream
- ½ cup white wine
- 2 tablespoons Dijon mustard
- 1 tomato peeled and chopped
- 1 tablespoons capers

Directions

i. Prepare the beef by shaping it to form 6 patties

ii. Put the butter into a skillet and heat it on medium-high heat.

iii. Add the onion plus garlic into the skillet and sauté for about 30 seconds to soften.

iv. Use salt and pepper to season the beef patties you prepared earlier, then add to the skillet and cook until it's done to your preferred degree. Turn it ones and when done, keep it aside but make sure it stays warm.

v. On the same skillet, cook the mushrooms so that they are done to preferably extent or until it turns brownish then add them to the warm patties prepared earlier.

vi. Take the mustard, the cream, tomato plus capers then heat them to the point where it heats up but not to boil.

vii. The mustard sauce can be used over the beef and mushrooms when serving.

https://www.ketodietyum.com/keto-beef-patties-with-creamy-mustard-sauce/

SHRIMP & ARTICHOKE PLATE

Servings 12

Calories 928

Fat 80 g

Proteins36 g

Carbs 7 g

Fiber 7 g

Sugar 2 g

Ingredients

- 24 eggs
- 60 ounce of cooked and peeled shrimp
- 75 ounces canned artichokes
- 36 sun-dried tomatoes in oil
- 3 cups mayonnaise
- 8 ½ ounces baby spinach
- 1.5 cups olive oil
- Salt and pepper

Directions

i. Place the eggs in already boiling water to cook for 4-8 minutes depending on whether you like them soft or hard-boiled.

ii. Cool the eggs in cold water for easier removal of the shell.

iii. Then place eggs, shrimp, artichokes, mayonnaise, sun-dried tomatoes, and spinach on a plate.

iv. Lastly, drizzle olive oil over the spinach. Season the taste with salt and pepper and serve.

https://www.dietdoctor.com/recipes/keto-shrimp-artichoke-plate

CORN DOG MUFFINS

Servings 20

Calories 78

Fat 7g

Proteins 2g

Carbs 1g

Sugar 0g

Ingredients

- ½ cup of blanched almond flour
- ½ cup flaxseed meal
- 1 tablespoon husk powder
- 3 tablespoons sweetener
- ¼ teaspoon salt
- ¼ teaspoon baking powder
- ¼ cup butter, melted
- 1 large egg
- 1/3 cup sour cream
- ¼ cup of coconut milk
- 3 hot dogs

Directions

i. Prepare the oven by preheating to 375 Fahrenheit.

ii. Take a large bowl and mix all the dry ingredients in it. Mix them well with the egg, sour cream, milk from the coconut and butter.

iii. Grease 20 mini-muffin slots then fill them with the batter. Slice the hot dogs into considerable sizes and place a peace at the middle of each muffin.

iv. Use the preheated oven for cooking them for relatively 12 minutes then broil them for another two minutes so that the tops are turning into a light brown.

v. Allow the muffins first to cool then transfer them on a wire rack so that they can completely cool down.

vi. Use some mayonnaise, chili paste and ketchup to make a dipping sauce.

vii. Enjoy them, especially for breakfast.

https://ketofiedsisters.com/keto-corn-dog-muffins/

ASIAN BEEF SALAD

Servings 4

Calories 355

Fat 20g

Proteins 30g

Carbs 13g

Fiber 3g

Sugar 4g

Ingredients

Marinade

- 2 Tablespoon fish sauce
- 2 tablespoon coconut aminos
- 2 tablespoon fresh lime juice
- 1 table spoon grated fresh ginger
- 1 large clove garlic, pressed and minced
- ¼ teaspoon chilli pepper flakes
- 1 tablespoon toasted sesame oil
- 1 pound sirloin steaks.

Salad

- 5 cups mixed lettuce
- 1 cup broccoli slaw
- 1 red bell pepper
- 4 ounces mushrooms
- 5 green onions, sliced thinly
- ¼ cup chopped cilantro
- 2 tablespoons sliced, toasted almond
- 2 tablespoons toasted sesame seed

Dressing

- 1 table spoon rice wine vinegar
- 2 tablespoons sunflower oil

Directions

i. Mix the marinade ingredients into a bowl without sirloin steak.

ii. Take the steak and place it in the marinade and turn the meat both sides so that it is well coated. Use a plastic wrap to cover then place it in the refrigerator so that to marinate for 2 hours or even overnight.

iii. Prepare the grill and make sure it heats with a medium-high temperature.

iv. Transfer the pre-prepared sirloin steak onto the grill and cook for about 4 minutes then turn the other side and grill for the same 4 minutes. It is well prepared if it achieves a golden brown color.

v. Place the steaks on to a plate then use a foil to cover then let it rest for about 10 minutes.

vi. On the side, take the lettuce, bell pepper, mushrooms, green onions, broccoli slaw, and cilantro into a bowl.

vii. On the other side, use the remaining marinade by pouring into a pan then simmer it for 5 minutes. Place the mixture aside then add vinegar and oil, ensuring you are stirring then place it aside.

viii. Slice the steak thinly while placing then gently on the salad.

ix. Serve the meal in four plates then use the toasted almonds and toasted sesame to dress.

x. Enjoy it as a homemade lunch for four.

https://cookingwithcurls.com/2019/01/24/asian-beef-salad/

AVOCADO, BACON AND GOAT CHEESE SALAD

Servings 4

Calories 1251

Fat 129g

Proteins 27g

Carbs 6g

Fiber 9g

Sugar 0g

Ingredients

- 8 ounces goat cheese
- 8 ounces bacon
- 2 avocados
- 4 ounces arugula lettuce
- 4 ounces walnuts
- 1 tablespoon lemon, the juice
- ½ cup mayonnaise
- ½ cup olive oil
- 2 tablespoon whipping cream
- Salt and pepper to taste

Directions

i.   Prepare the oven first. Heat it to 400 degrees Fahrenheit then prepare a baking dish by placing a parchment paper.

ii.   Slice the cheese so that it is in small rounds about half an inch and place them on the baking dish. Place it in the upper rank of the oven and bake on the top rack until they turn golden.

iii.   Prepare the bacon on a pan by frying it until it is a bit crispy.

iv.   Take the avocado to prepare it by cutting it into small pieces that can be used to top arugula. Now take the bacon plus goat cheese and add to it as you top with sprinkled nuts.

v.   Take the lemon, mayonnaise, olive, and the cream and use an immersion blender to prepare a paste. Add salt and pepper to season and use it for dressing the meal.

vi.   Serve it and enjoy with friends for brunch.

https://www.dietdoctor.com/recipes/avocado-bacon-goat-cheese-salad

SMOKED SALMON PLATE

Servings 5

Calories 1403

Fat 109%

Proteins 105grams

Carbs 1grams

Fiber 1gram

Sugar 3 g

Ingredients

- 2 pounds smoked salmon
- 2 ½ cups of mayonnaise
- 5 1/3 ounces baby spinach
- 2 ½ tablespoon olive oil
- 1 ¼ limes
- Salt and pepper

Directions

i.   Put salmon, spinach, and a wedge in a plate. Scoop the mayonnaise and lime and spread on the meal.

ii.   Take the olive oil and drizzle over the meal then season using salt and pepper.

iii.   Serve in five portions.

https://www.dietdoctor.com/recipes/keto-smoked-salmon-plate/serving/5

TORTILLA WITH GROUND BEEF & SALSA

Servings 4

Calories 822

Fat 67g

Proteins 42g

Carbs 8g

Fiber 10g

Ingredients

For Tortilla & Beef

- 2 eggs
- 2 egg whites
- 2 ounces cream cheese, softened
- ½ teaspoon salt
- 1½ teaspoon ground pysllium husk powder
- 1 tablespoon coconut flour
- 2 tablespoon olive oil
- 1 pound of ground beef, at room temperature
- 2 tablespoon Tex-Mex seasoning
- ½ cup water
- Salt and pepper
- 6 ounces shredded Mexican cheese
- 3 ounces shredded lettuce

For Salsa

- 2 avocados diced
- 1 tomato, diced
- 2 tbsp lime juice
- 1 tbsp olive oil
- ½ cup fresh cilantro, chopped
- Salt and pepper

Directions

i. Prepare the oven first by preheating it until you achieve 200 degrees Celsius (400 degrees Fahrenheit).

ii. Use a whisk and beat the eggs and the egg white for a few minutes until you achieve the fluffy solution. Use a separate bowl to prepare the cheese by beating it until you reach the smoothness needed. Add the eggs to the cheese then continue whisking until you have achieved a smooth batter.

iii. Put the salt, psyllium and coconut flour into a bowl then mix with batter one spoon at a time while whisking. When the dough is well mixed, it is necessary to allow it rest to swell.

iv. Using two baking sheets, cover them with parchment paper one at a time then take the batter and spread it thinly on each using a spatula forming at least 4 circles.

v. Place the sheet into the oven top rack then bake for 5 minutes or use the change of edges to brown to tell they are cooked. Make sure you confirm that the bottom side is not burning.

vi. On the side, prepare the grounded beef by frying on a pan with oil at medium-high heat.

vii. Add to it the seasoning then water and stir for some time before leaving it to simmer for some minute until the water is gone.

Preparing Salsa

viii. Take the avocado, lime juice, tomatoes, olive, and cilantro to prepare the salsa making sure they are well seasoned with salt and pepper.

ix. Use the tortilla, shredded cheese, salsa, and lettuce to serve the beef filling.

https://www.dietdoctor.com/recipes/keto-tortilla-ground-beef-salsa

ASIAN CABBAGE STIR-FRY

Servings 4

Calories 1139

Fat 97g

Proteins 48g

Carbs 18g

Fiber 4.5g

Sugar 8g

Proteins 48g

Ingredients

- ¾Kg Green Cabbage
- 142gm Vegan Butter
- ½Kg beef, skirt steak
- 1 tablespoon Salt
- 1 tablespoon Onion powder
- ¼ tablespoon black pepper (ground)
- 1 tablespoon white wine vinegar
- 2 clove(s) garlic
- 3 tablespoon green onion, scallion, ramp
- 1 tablespoon korean red chili flakes
- 1 tablespoon ginger, ground (fresh; finely chopped or grated)
- 1 tablespoon sesame oil
- 1 cup mayonnaise
- ½ tablespoon wasabi paste

Directions

i. Using a knife to shred the cabbage into fine sizes (a food processor will also do the work).

ii. Take at least 3 ounces of the butter and fry the cabbage until they are soft enough but do not allow them to turn brown.

iii. Pour into the cabbage the spices then allow them to simmer for some few minutes while stirring then server the cabbage into a bowl.

iv. Put the remaining butter into the frying pan then melt adding into it the garlic, chili and ginger then cook for about three minutes.

v. Add into the mixture the grounded meat and cook until it is well prepared and the meat loses all the juice through evaporation. Reduce the heat for the remaining process.

vi. Take the cabbage, and the scallions then add it to the meat and mix them through until everything is hot. Use the salt and pepper to season according to favorable taste top the meal with sesame oil.

vii. Prepare on the side mayonnaise by mixing it with wasabi until you achieve the right flavor.

viii. Take the stir fry and serve it while warm and top it with wasabi mayonnaise.

ROAST BEEF & CHEDDAR

Servings 2

Calories 1071

Fat 98g

Proteins 38g

Carbs 6g

Fiber 8g

Ingredients

7 ounces deli roast beef

5 ounces cheddar cheese

1 avocado

6 radishes

1 scallion

½ cup mayonnaise

1 tablespoon Dijon mustard

2 ounces lettuce

2 tablespoon olive oil

Salt and pepper

Directions

i.   Take a dry clean plate and on it place the roast beef, cheddar cheese, avocado plus radishes.

ii. Pic the sliced onions and arrange them with mustard plus a well-arranged dollop of mayonnaise.

iii. Use the lettuce to serve and lightly pour the olive oil on top,

iv. Season the meal with salt and pepper, and it is ready to eat for breakfast.

PESTO CHICKEN CASSEROLE

Servings 10

Calories 1018

Fat 93 g

Proteins 38 g

Carbs 6 g

Fiber 2 g

Sugar 3 g

Ingredients

- 1.7 kgs boneless chicken thighs
- Salt and pepper
- 5 tablespoons better/coconut oil
- 13tbspn red pesto
- 225 gram pitted olives
- 350 grams feta cheese
- 2 ½ garlic cloves

Directions

i. Preheat the oven to 400 degrees Fahrenheit

ii. Slice the chicken so that you have bite sizes and use salt and pepper to season.

iii. Using a large skillet, take butter and fry the chicken pieces into batches on medium heat until golden brown.

iv. Take a bowl and mix pesto and heavy cream.

v. When the chicken is ready fried, place in a baking dish.

vi. Take the olives, feta cheese, and garlic and add to the chicken in the dish. Add the pesto.

vii. Use the oven to bake for roughly 25 minutes until the dish turns bubbly and light brown around the edges.

viii. When its ready server into ten portions.

https://www.dietdoctor.com/recipes/keto-pesto-chicken-casserole/servings/10

COCONUT PORRIDGE

Servings 6

Calories 303

Fat 25g

Proteins 3g

Carbs 17g

Fiber 11g

Sugar 1g

Ingredients

- 1 cup shredded coconut

- 2 cups coconut milk
- 1 2/3 cups water
- ¼ cup coconut flour
- ¼ cup whole psyllium husks
- 1 teaspoon vanilla extract
- ½ teaspoon cinnamon
- ¼ teaspoon nutmeg
- 30 drops stevia liquid
- 20 drops monk fruit liquid

Directions

i. Place a pot on a medium-high hot heater then toast the coconut until you achieve a golden look and stay alert that it does not burn.

ii. Add the coconut milk together with milk and stir carefully.

iii. Use a covering and bring the meal to a boiling point.

iv. Transfer the pot away from the heat or turn the heat off then open the lid remaining careful of the steam.

v. Add the remaining ingredients and stir the mixture thoroughly.

vi. Serve in a porridge bowl and enjoy for breakfast.

https://lowcarbyum.com/coconut-low-carb-porridge-instant-pot/

WAGON WHEEL SAUSAGE PIE

Servings 2

Calories 386

Fat 17g

Proteins 17g

Carbs 44g

Fiber 3g

Sugar 4g

Ingredients

- 1½ cups of frozen and shredded potatoes, thawed
- 3 tablespoons cream cheese, softened
- 2 tablespoons plus 2 teaspoons 2% milk, divided
- 1 green onion, chopped

- 1/8 teaspoon salt, optional
- Dash pepper
- 4 uncooked breakfast sausages links
- ¼ cup biscuit/ baking mix
- 1 large egg
- Dash ground nutmeg
- Dash paprika

Directions

i. Take a pie plate about 7 inches, and coat with cooking spray then place the hash browns.

ii. On the side, take the small bowl and mix the cheese, milk, onions, salt, and pepper thoroughly. Later spread the potatoes over.

iii. Slice the sausages into halves then place them over the potatoes arranging them in spoke-like design.

iv. Use another small bowl then mix the biscuit with eggs nutmeg and milk leftover so that to attain the smooth mixture. Pour the mixture in between the sausages then use the paprika to sprinkle appropriately.

v. Place the pate in a preheated oven in 400 degrees Fahrenheit for about 25 minutes so that they turn golden brown.

vi. Take the meal from the oven and allow it to rest for some time, then serve while still warm for breakfast.

https://www.tasteofhome.com/recipes/wagon-wheel-breakfast-pie/

CHINESE BEEF STIR-FRY WITH ORANGE

Servings 1

Calories 649

Fat 44.5g

Proteins 53.5g

Carbs 2g

Fiber 0g

Ingredients

3.5 ounces of beef thinly slice

¼ cup beef broth

1 tablespoon coconut oil

½ medium onion diced

2 medium green onions thinly sliced

¼ orange zest and juice

2 cloves garlic minced

1 inch ginger sliced

1 pinch ground cinnamon

½ teaspoon soy sauce

½ teaspoon fish sauce

1 Bay Leaf

Directions

i. Cut the beef into thin slices and dice the onion into favorable sizes.

ii. Place an iron skillet on the heat and add coconut oil then cook the onions, garlic plus ginger for one minute.

iii. Add the beef to cook of another 5 minutes. On it add soy, fish sauce, bay leaf, cinnamon and also orange juice plus the beef broth.

iv. Increase the heating and continue cooking so that there is a thickened juice.

v. The meal should now be ready to serve in a plate while sprinkled with the orange zest plus some green onions.

https://www.ketodietyum.com/keto-stir-fried-beef-with-orange/

BEEF & PUMPKIN HASH

Servings 4

Calories 763

Fat 61g

Proteins 43g

Carbs 8g

Fiber 1g

Sugar 3g

Ingredients

- 800g beef, minced
- 500g pumpkin
- 250g bacon, organic
- 3-4 tablespoons fresh parsley
- 3 tablespoons ghee or butter

- 1 tablespoon paprika
- ½ teaspoon cayenne pepper
- Pinch freshly ground black pepper
- ¼ teaspoon salt

Directions

i. Prepare the pumpkin by cutting into half then removing the seeds.

ii. On the side, have the beef in a bowl in room temperature awaiting preparation.

iii. Peel off the outer cover of the pumpkin then dice it into small cubes

iv. Grease a pan with ghee and then cook the pumpkin in it making sure that they cook well from all sides. Allow the meal to cook for roughly 10 minutes, making sure that you stir at least twice to prevent them from burning.

v. Prepare on the side by slicing and then roasting them in a pan until they are brownish.

vi. Take the spices and mix with minced meat in a bowl. Once ready, place it in a greased pan with ghee and cook so that to attain the brown look and make sure the meat is well stirred.

vii. Add to it the crispy bacon prepared early and thoroughly mix adding to them the cooked parsley.

viii. Add to the combination the sautéed pumpkin and mix well then serve in plates while garnished with parsley.

https://ketodietapp.com/Blog/lchf/Pumpkin-Beef-Sautee

JALAPEÑOS POPPER BALLS

Servings 12

Calories 305

Fat 20g

Proteins 14g

Carbs 15g

Fiber 0g

Sugar 2g

Ingredients

- 2 cups panko breadcrumbs
- 2 cups shredded cheddar cheese
- 2 large eggs
- 1 teaspoon kosher salt

- 1 teaspoon black pepper
- 10 ounces cream cheese
- 4 cooked stripped bacon
- 4 jalapeños

Directions

i. Put the bread crumbs, eggs, cheddar cheese, ½ teaspoon pepper, and ½ teaspoon salt in a bowl and mix thoroughly.

ii. Take nonstick spray and grease a muffin of 24-cup capacity and heap every cup with at least a tablespoon of the mixture. Press the fillings well so that they are firmly placed in the pan. Place the tin aside.

iii. Using another bowl, take the cream cheese, bacon, jalapeños, the remaining salt, and pepper then combine them well.

iv. While doing these, prepare the oven to preheat up to 375 degrees Fahrenheit.

v. Take the cream cheese mixture, and ill at least two tablespoons of the crumb wells prepared earlier, then top with the cheddar and jalapeños slices.

vi. Place the tin into the oven to cook for 10 minutes. When they are golden brown, then they are ready.

vii. Enjoy them, especially for breakfast.

https://tasty.co/recipe/jalapeno-popper-bites

CARBONARA

Servings 4

Calories 373

Fat 8grams

Proteins 11grams

Carbs 3 grams

Fiber 3grams

Sugar 1 ½ grams

Ingredients

- 2 ounces of salted butter
- 7 ounces of bacon, diced
- I clove of garlic, finely chopped
- ½ teaspoon of pepper

- 1 pound of cauliflower, cut in to small florets
- ¾ cup of heavy cream
- ½ cup of parmesan cheese shaved
- I egg yolk

Directions

i. Cook bacon and garlic in a non-stick frying pan for 3-5 minutes over medium heat until the bacon turns brown.

ii. Add pepper and cauliflower and stir well - cook for 3 minutes.

iii. With reduced heat to low add cream. Go on with the cooking so that the cream has a thick appearance and the cauliflower is tender.

iv. Turn off heat and add the parmesan and egg yolk then whisk stir the meal.

v. Once well combined, serve in 4 bowls.

https://www.myketokitchen.com/keto-recipes/one-pan-low-card-cauliflower-carbonara/

BAKED BACON OMELET

Servings 6

Calories 737

Fat 72 g

Proteins 21g

Carbs 2 g

Fiber 1 g

Sugar1 g

Ingredients

- 12 eggs
- 15 ounces bacon(cubes)
- 9 ounces butter
- 60 ounces fresh spinach
- 3 tablespoon finely chopped fresh chives
- Salt and pepper
- 30 grams cheddar cheese

Directions

i. Preheat the oven to 400 degrees Fahrenheit.

ii. With butter, grease the baking dish.

iii. Use the remaining butter to fry the spinach together with bacon in a separate dish.

iv. Whisk the eggs. Mix the spinach and bacon, cheddar cheese, and use the leftover fat to do the fry.

v. Take the chopped chives and season with the salt plus pepper.

vi. Pour the egg mixture in the baking dish and bake for 20 minutes until set and golden brown.

vii. Let it cool and serve.

https://www.dietdoctor.com/recipes/keto-baked-bacon-omelet

PANCAKES WITH BERRIES AND WHIPPED CREAM

Servings 6

Calories 425

Fat 39 g

Proteins 13 g

Carbs 5 g

Fiber 3 g

Sugar 0

Ingredients

- 6 eggs
- 300 grams cottage cheese
- 12 grams ground psyllium husk powder
- 75 grams butter/coconut oil.
- 1 scoop keto protein powder vanilla
- 175 ml fresh rasp berries or fresh blue berries
- 350 ml heavy whipping cream
- 50 ml-100 ml sugar free maple syrup

Directions

i. Take the eggs and mix with cottage cheese, and ground psyllium husk and protein powder in a medium-sized bowl. Allow it to rest for about 8 minutes so that to achieve the necessary thickness.

ii. Heat the butter in a non-stick skillet — Fry pancakes on medium heat for 3-4 minutes on each side.

iii. Then add heavy whipping to a separate bowl and whip it until soft peaks form.

iv. Serve the pancakes — best for breakfast.

https://ketoconnection.com.au/sweet-keto-pancakes-with-berries-whipped-cream/

FRITTATA WITH FRESH SPINACH

Servings 4

Calories 280

Fat 22g

Proteins 18g

Carbs 5g

Sugar 2g

Fiber 1.7g

Ingredients

- 9 large eggs
- 2 tablespoon milk
- 1/3 cup parmesan cheese grated
- ¼ teaspoon salt
- 1/8 teaspoon ground pepper, fresh
- 2 tablespoon extra-virgin olive oil
- 1 medium onion, chopped
- 1 large clove garlic, minced
- Sun dried tomatoes, 2 tablespoon chopped
- 8 ounces fresh spinach, chopped
- 2 ounces goat cheese

Directions

i. Put the eggs, parmesan, milk, salt, and pepper in a bowl and whisk them together to mix well.

ii. Pour the olive oil to a skillet at a medium temperature. Add into it the onion and sauté so that it achieves the translucent look. Take the garlic and pour together with tomatoes then cook it in a minute or so.

iii. Take the spinach in handful and add to the cooking onions making sure you mix using tongs. Continue adding as they wilt until all of them are fully cooked to your preference. They shouldn't get too soft.

iv. Pour the egg mixture into the cooking spinach and make sure it is evenly spread to the bottom.

v. Take the cheese and sprinkle over on top of the frittata.

vi. Lower the heat to the lowest level then allow it to cook for relatively 10 to 13 minutes so that all the center of the meal is set.

vii. Broil the frittata in an oven for another 3 minutes then remove when the golden color forms.

viii. Let it rest with oven mitts on it and allow it cool for some minutes.

ix. It is well serve when sliced into wedges while still warm.

https://www.simplyrecipes.com/recipes/spinach_frittata/

FRIED SALMON WITH BROCCOLI & CHEESE

Servings 12

Calorie 684

Fat 52 g

Proteins 46 g

Carbs 6 g

Fiber 3g

Sugar 2g

Ingredients

- 3 pounds broccoli
- 9 ounce butter
- Salt and pepper
- 15 ounce grated cheddar cheese
- 4 ½ punds salmon
- 3 limes

Directions

i. Preheat the oven to 400 degrees Fahrenheit.

ii. Cut the broccolis into smaller florets. Simmer them in water that is lightly salted for some minutes. The broccoli should maintain a texture that is chewable and the original colored.

iii. Remove the broccoli from the water and ensure that they are thoroughly drained. Set aside and allow the steam to evaporate.

iv. Place the broccoli in a well-greased baking dish. Add butter and pepper to taste.

v. Sprinkle cheese on top the broccoli and bake in the oven for 15-20 minutes until cheese turns a golden color.

vi. Use the salt and pepper to season the salmon and fry in plenty of butter.

vii. Serve it in 12 portions.

ZUCCHINI HASH BROWNS

Servings 6

Calories 45

Fat 2g

Proteins 3g

Carbs 2g

Fiber 1g

Sugar 1g

Ingredients

- 2 zucchinis
- Salt, to taste
- ½ cup parmesan cheese grated
- 15 grams fresh chives
- 1 teaspoon dried oregano
- ¼ teaspoon garlic powder
- ¼ teaspoon black pepper
- 1 egg

Directions

i. Switch on the oven and heat in first to 400 degrees Fahrenheit.

ii. Take the zucchini and grate it on the side then transfer grated one into a large bowl.

iii. Sprinkle some salt and mix them until well done then allow it to rest for 20 minutes. The salt will draw moisture from it during the rest.

iv. Use a kitchen towel to squeeze the excess liquid from the zucchini into another bowl and put them back to the original container.

v. Toss into it chives, garlic powder, parmesan, oregano, black pepper and then the egg then thoroughly mix so that they are well combined.

vi. Make about 6 portions of the zucchini mixture and create some patties using a well-lined baking sheet.

vii. Place them into the oven and bake them for 35 minutes to attain a golden brown look.

viii. Allow the hash browns to cool for down for about 10 minutes to be well set.

ix. Prepare a dipping source that is to your preference end enjoy for breakfast.

MINI CRUSTLESS QUICHES

Calories: 382

Fat 28

Proteins 22

Carbs 5.3

Ingredients

- 6 Large eggs

- 3 Plum tomatoes, diced

- 2/3 Cup mozzarella cheese, shredded

- 1/3 Cup pepper jack cheese, shredded

- 1/3 Cup sweet onion, diced

- 1/3 Cup sliced pickled jalapenos

- 2/3 Cup soppressata salami, diced

- 1/3 Cup heavy cream

Directions

i. Prepare the oven first by preheating it to 325 degrees Fahrenheit then grease a 15" X 11" muffin tin.

ii. Place the ingredients in a mixing bowl, season with salt and pepper and whisk well.

iii. Divide the paste in muffin tins making sure the batter is equal than bake them in the oven for 25 minutes.

iv. Wait for them to cool down then store them in the fridge. You can eat them whenever ready by reheating them.

v. The ingredients above should be enough to prepare 4 Mini Crustless Quiches

vi.   The meal is ideal when taken during breakfast.

TUNA AVOCADO SALAD

Calories: 508

Fats 34g

Proteins 31g

Carbs 5

Ingredients

- 4 Ounces of canned tuna

- ½ Stalk celery, diced

- ½ Avocado

- 2 Tablespoon mayonnaise

- 1 Teaspoon mustard

- ½ Teaspoon fresh lemon juice

- Salt, pepper

- 1 Hard-boiled egg, peeled, chopped

Directions

i.   Combine the tuna celery and avocado.

ii.   Add mayo, mustard lemon juice, and spices.

iii.   Add the egg to the tuna salad

iv.   Mix the combination until the ingredients are well blended.

v.   You can pack it and have it for lunch.

https://www.tasteaholics.com/pdf/14-day-meal-plan.pdf?utm_campaign=mass-email&utm_source=email&utm_medium=newsletter